Ketogenic Diet Book for Beginners

30-Day Quick Start Guide
To Losing Weight Fast

By Coral James

Table of Contents

Introduction

We live in a world where there are 101 different ways to lose weight. From protein shakes to detoxes or simply working out, it can be difficult to know which one to do and if any of them really work. Maybe you have heard that the best weight to lose weight is on a Paleo Diet or the Gluten free diet. But the truth is there are many ways to lose weight but...... the Ketogenic diet is the easiest and most satisfying way to lose weight and FAST! And there are other so many other health benefits; limiting and preventing heart disease and epilepsy while the increased energy will make you feel amazing. In this book you are going to learn how to avoid the common mistakes that most people make and how to lose weight fast in 30 days on a Ketogenic Diet. So far in your life, if you have been unable to lose weight on "diets" then look no more, this book is for you. Get the body you have always wanted now, so let's get started.

Chapter 1 – The History of Ketogenic Diet & What is Ketogenic Diet

The Ketogenic diet has been used in the treatment of different clinical conditions over the years including childhood epilepsy. Research indicates that in the middle ages, fasting was used as a remedy for seizures. In the early 1900's, seizures in children were treated by fasting. However, it turned out that fasting was not as effective as the experts once thought. Therefore, they attempted to discover a better method to mimic starvation Ketosis while at the same time consuming food.

According to research, a diet low in carbohydrates, minimal levels of protein and high in fat could maintain starvation Ketosis for long periods of time. It was not long before these findings gave way to the introduction of the Ketogenic diet in 1921 by Doctor Wilder. This diet was able to control pediatric epilepsy in situations where drugs as well as other remedies had previously failed. Dr. Wilder's Ketogenic diet is significantly indistinguishable from the diet used in 1988 to manage childhood epilepsy.

During the 1930's, 1940's and 1950's, the Ketogenic diet fell into insignificance due to the development of a new epilepsy treatment. The diet lost its appeal from then on as prescription drugs seemed to be the easier option. A number of modified Ketogenic diets were trialled, but they all fell into obscurity. Later in 1992, the story of Charlie (a 2-year old with epilepsy) rediscovered the Ketogenic diet, since the child's condition could not be treated with medication.

Charlie began the Ketogenic diet and in a matter of weeks he had responded remarkably well. This encouraged Charlie's father to begin the Charlie Foundation. The foundation educates and promotes the Ketogenic diet. This resulted in a great number of medical centers to start recommending the Ketogenic diet and a number of detailed studies have proven its effectiveness.

Based on its history, the Ketogenic diet requires the dieter to be informed and stay committed in order to initiate and maintain the program. The best outcomes are obtained when the progress of the diet is monitored by a team of specialists. The diet requires commitment by the families of the people undertaking the diet, and ongoing medical advice and support by the treatment team. Epilepsy is to date the medical condition that has been treated and managed the most using the Ketogenic diet.

What is the Ketogenic Diet?

The Ketogenic diet is a high-fat diet that induces physiological changes, which mimics periods of fasting or starvation. What the diet simply does is switch the bodies energy source from glucose to Ketone bodies – well known as nutritional Ketosis. The Ketogenic diet is made up of 80% to 90% of calories that are primarily obtained from fat. The protein content ranges from 50g to 80g per day; however, it is less carbohydrates (10g to 20g per day).

Types of Ketogenic Diet

1. Classic Ketogenic Diet

The classic Ketogenic diet was created in the 1920s and it is low in carbohydrates, adequate in protein and high in fat. The classic Ketogenic diet utilizes long chain triglycerides. It usually takes 24 to 72 hours to fast to the moment Ketosis is achieved. The use of long chain triglycerides is at 3:1 or 4:1 of the caloric intake throughout Ketosis. This diet was originally created to mimic the effects of starvation; however, the classic Ketogenic diet was engaged less frequently after the discovery of phenytoin. The fats in the classic Ketogenic diet are made up of a mixture plant-derived fats and animal fat; and fatty acids of variable chain length are normally included. As a result, the classic Ketogenic diet contains plenty of saturated fatty acids.

2. Modified Ketogenic Diet

The modified Ketogenic diet is based on a high protein, low carb and middling vegetable diet. It uses medium chain triglycerides to cause gastric upset. This diet is more pleasant and allows the dieter to engage more non-Ketogenic foods. The modified Ketogenic diet is based on identical principles of medium chain triglyceride and classic Ketogenic diets. In simple terms, the modified Ketogenic diet has high fat and low amounts of carbohydrates. This means that modified KD has the same effects as classic and medium chain triglyceride as far as changing the balance of energy production fuels is concerned. This diet actually uses fat for energy instead of glucose.

3. Radcliffe Infirmary Diet

This diet uses a mixture of long chain triglycerides and medium chain triglycerides. It is considered a variant, but calories are not limited since the dieter can limit carbohydrates to 10 to 20 grams per day. Basically, the Radcliffe infirmary diet is a cyclic as well as targeted Ketogenic diet.

Why the Ketogenic Diet?

The Ketogenic diet is based on low-carb principles, and low-carb diets are popular for the benefits they provide. Hunger is the greatest adversary of dieting, since most people give up dieting due to the overwhelming urge to eat. One of the positive aspects of the Ketogenic diet is to help in the reduction of appetite. KD's are much more helpful in losing weight when compared to low-fat diets.

The Ketogenic diet increases the levels of good cholesterol, HDL. Basically, LDL carries cholesterol from a dieter's liver to the rest of the body, while HDL carries cholesterol to the liver away from the body. This means that it can either be used or excreted by the liver; therefore, higher levels of HDL lower the risk of heart diseases. Research indicates that reducing carbs can significantly lead to a visible reduction of blood pressure and risk of many common ailments.

Ketogenic diets are individualized as well as structured regimes that provide particular meal plans. The diet require foods to be measured and they require meals to be ingested completely. Unlike other diets, the ratio of these diets can be effectively adjusted to result in better performance. Ketogenic diets are also considered to be low glycemic treatments, which lead to steady glucose levels. As far as Ketogenic diets are concerned, no liquids are restricted.

Facts About Ketogenic Diets

- Ketogenic diets require medical supervision.
- They are high in fat, medium in protein and low in carb.
- The ratio of fat to carb and protein in Ketogenic diets is 1:1, 2:1, 3:1, 4:1
- Food is weighed.
- Ketogenic diets use meal plans.
- They are normally started at the hospital.
- Calories are controlled.
- They require minerals, supplements and vitamins.
- These diets do not restrict fluids.

Chapter 2 –Benefits of Ketogenic Diet

A Ketogenic diet is a diet that is rich in fat, which contains acceptable amounts of proteins and low carbohydrates. The diet is basically used to manage epilepsy in children. However, the diet is nowadays considered to be highly effective in burning fats and shedding weight quickly and effectively. Usually, the carbs contained in food are transformed to glucose and then transported throughout the body. The Ketogenic diet however, leaves less carbs to be converted. This forces the liver to convert the fats stored in the body into fatty acids along with other Ketone bodies. The process is referred to as Ketosis. The Ketone bodies are the ones used as the energy source instead of glucose. Ketogenic diets are associated with many health benefits for the body.

Benefits of Ketogenic Diet

1. Reduces Appetite Naturally

One of the most amazing discoveries as far as Ketogenic diets are concerned is the ability to kill appetite of a dieter after a number of days. The KD diet increases Ketones, which is accompanied by an upsurge in Ghrelin. An increas in Ghrelin is usually observed in weight loss. People who lose weight via KD will also present with a significant decrease in the following: pancreatic polypeptide levels, amylin, peptide YY and leptin. Research indicates that dieters on KD have greatly reduced hunger. If your implementing the KD, you will feel more satisfied and slightly less hungry.

2. Ketogenic Diets are Much More Helpful in Losing Weight

KD's are significantly more effective as far as losing weight is concerned. Ketogenic diets are much more helpful in losing weight when compared to any other diet plan. These diets normally address and fix hormonal imbalance. The issue of hormonal imbalance is associated with symptoms of overeating and the lack of energy to workout. In simple words, if your insulin and blood sugar are imbalanced, you will feel hungry and overeat. Ketogenic diets ensure that the body is left with only option, that is to use the alternative source of energy instead of glucose.

3. Increases Levels of Good Cholesterol

Ketogenic diets increases levels of good cholesterol (HDL). HDL normally carries cholesterol to the liver away from the body; while LDL carries cholesterol from the liver to the rest of the body. The cholesterol can be used or excreted by the liver. On the other hand, the cholesterol carried to the body is stored in the body leading to health hazards. Therefore, higher levels of good cholesterol lower the risk of heart diseases. Research suggests that low carb intake can significantly lead to a perceptible reduction of blood pressure. As a result, a dieter will be less exposed to the various risks of common diseases, especially heart diseases.

Why Only 5% of Dieters Succeed

Only a handful of people succeed with KD because of common mistakes. Usually people do not give themselves enough time to adjust. Basically, some dieters try KD's for three to four days or a week, and when they feel like crap, they stop. These are the people who say they have tried Ketogenic diets, but they do not work. These people normally complain that their performance suffered and they could not function. However you must remember that it takes time to adjust to KD's. This is because you are completely changing your metabolism and your main source of energy. The major change is the energy source that fuels your body, and this takes time since you have never been in Ketosis before. If you have never been in a state of deep Ketosis, it will take you several weeks or months for you to experience the benefits of a Ketogenic diet. In the very beginning you will lose a little bit of weight really fast. During the induction phase, most people will feel good , but you have to realize that there may be a time when you should expect yourself to feel like crap. This can be anywhere between a few days to a few weeks. Not giving enough time for your body to catch up with a Ketogenic diet is a serious mistake made by most people attempting it.

The second biggest mistake people make, is the inability to know what they are doing from the very start. A lot of people jump into KD not knowing what types of foods to eat or what types of fats they prefer to eat. Instead they buy a whole bunch of coconut oil and MCT oil to fill their bellies, which will definitely upset the stomach. This approach is unsustainable and a suboptimal way to implement a Ketogenic diet. If you want to go on a KD, you need to make sure that you are getting all the micronutrients and macronutrients you need.

You need to ensure that you get enough fats in the beginning, because you do not want to just eat a little bit of protein and cut your calories to rock bottom. Eating less protein will not make you feel okay when starting a KD. In the beginning, it is advisable to not reduce it too much. When you go into too much of a deficit and you try to switch over to burning fats, you will just be giving your body a little bit of protein, which is just not an optimal scenario. You will not have enough calories for your body to feel satisfied, and your body will go into stress mode. Therefore, know what you are doing, eat enough calories, but do not drop your calories too low. This does not mean that you need to eat five sticks of butter with every meal, but just ensure they are not too low. Make sure your carbs are coming from leafy green vegetables. This is an important aspect to consider, as you do not want to waste your carbs on foods that your body does not require.

This simply means that everything you eat in a KD should have a purpose; either towards meeting your micronutrient goals, getting fibre in, or providing your gut with beneficial bacteria. There should be a purpose for every food you eat; and therefore everything should be beneficial. When you start a KD the foods are very nutrient dense or very caloric, but they do not take up a lot of space in your body. To ensure that you make as few mistakes as possible, you need to do a lot of research before tackling the KD head-on. If you have friends who have been on a Ketogenic diets for a long time, talk to them about it. This will allow you to figure out what kind of food they are eating and what kind of foods they like. Do not just assume that it will be easy; give yourself at least a little bit of variety. Make sure that your diet involves simple meals and consistency.

This does not mean that you should conveniently settle for bacon and eggs, since there are other potential sources of macronutrients, such as fish and seafood. Widen your horizons and figure out what foods you like, because these will be your fat sources. Use carbs wisely. Don't eat two bites of a pop tart for your thirty grams of carbs. Be smart and make every single calorie count in your Ketogenic Diet plan.

Chapter 3 – In Depth Look at Ketosis & Ketogenic Diets

Ketosis has many benefits. To best understand KD's, you need to know exactly what the Ketosis process involves. Ketosis is an abnormal increase of Ketone bodies in the blood. What is referred to as lipid metabolism remains intact when a dieter's body is in a Ketogenic state. As a result, the body will embark on breaking down body fat to provide fuel to promote the body's normal functions.

Ketosis increases the dieter's body aptitude to use fats to fuel the body's functions instead of carbs. When one is consuming high amount of carbs, the body adapts to a routine energy source. However, things change when the Ketogenic diet is introduced. The body has to adapt to using fats as far as fuelling the body is concerned. Generally, KD's use more fats for energy in place of carbs. Ketosis in conjunction with a considerable protein intake does effectively suppress appetite. This is so since the dieter has to ingest a large amount of fat for the diet to be effective as a KD. The process of Ketosis spares protein, and that's why the Ketogenic diet involves medium amounts of proteins. When undertaking a KD, the dieter's body will prefer Ketones instead of glucose. The large amounts of fats present in the body mean that the body does not have to oxidize proteins in order to produce glucose. Ketosis ensures that the body's insulin levels are low. As a result, the body experiences free-glycerol release and greater lipolysis when compared to a normal diet. Increased insulin levels prohibit the body from using fatty acids to fuel the body's function. Low insulin level promotes the release of growth hormone.

So far you have come across the word Ketone or a Ketone body. A Ketone body is simply what is formed when fatty acids are converted in to fuel. The Ketone bodies include acetone, acetoacetate, and β-hydroxybutyrate. These Ketone bodies can be utilized by any body tissue that contains mitochondria, such as the brain and muscle. To be able to maintain the KD you will need to understand the following principles;

1. Fat Intake

To understand correctly the amount of fat you need to take in your KD you first need to know the different kinds of fats. Basically, there are three major kinds of fats; trans fats, unsaturated fats and saturated fats. In most cases, most dieters who undertake KD's fail to understand the concept behind each type of fat. Normally, saturated fats are known to be bad fats for the body, but the problem arises when a dieter cannot differentiate this from unsaturated fats. Fats are categorized with respect to their chemical structure. Therefore, whether a fat molecule is unsaturated or saturated depends primarily on the number of hydrogen atoms contained in the molecule. Usually, saturated fats are obtained from animal products, such as cheese, milk, eggs and meat. The Ketogenic diet will require you to consume at least a reasonable amount of saturated fat. This seems to alarm a great number of people using the KD for the first time. Most people's concerns have to do with cardiovascular disorders and atherosclerosis associated with saturated fats. Nonetheless, saturated fat and all the diseases and conditions linked to it should not concern you too much. This is so since KD allows your body to burn a huge amount of fat in a single day through Ketosis. This simply means that the saturated fat will not stay in your body for a long time before the body converts it into energy. This is the main reason why an abnormal fat intake is encouraged in KD.

Unsaturated fats are primarily obtained from plant sources. Unsaturated fats are considered to be healthier and most diets that people engage will recommend them over saturated fats. However, there is one major problem with these sources (plants), and this is the high carbohydrate content. This simply means that it can be difficult to balance carb avoidance and the intake of unsaturated fat. The best way to get around this problem is to settle for unsaturated fat sources that have low amounts of carbohydrates, such as olive oil and flax oil.

Trans-fat on the other hand is a fatty acid that has been produced by hydrogenating an unsaturated fatty acid (and so changing its shape), found in processed foods such as margarine and fried foods and puddings and commercially baked goods and partially hydrogenated vegetable oils. A great number of dieters do not know that trans-fats also occur naturally in extremely small amounts and the body can easily deal with. Nonetheless, man-made trans-fats are usually found in high amounts, particularly in processed foods. These processed foods as mentioned earlier include margarine and fried foods and puddings and commercially baked goods and partially hydrogenated vegetable oils. Trans-fats, particularly man-made have been associated with health issues such as coronary heart disease. As long as you are obtaining the correct amount of calories, ingesting enough protein while limiting carb intake, then the rest of the calories will be obtained from fats through Ketosis. The only trick is to ensure that the high amount of fat you are consuming comes from high quality sources, such as cold-water fish, flax oil, coconut oil and any other unprocessed food.

2. Protein Intake

The fact that you will be tremendously reducing the amount of carbs you ingest means that you have to increase your fat and protein intake. There is a dilemma as far as protein is concerned, because ingesting less protein will leave the body with less calories and ingesting too much protein will inhibit Ketosis. This is so since the body will first burn the calories in the extra protein before converting fat in to Ketone bodies. Your protein intake should be based on two aspects: sedentary level and active level. Ingesting less protein can be detrimental to a dieter's weight loss campaign and his or her general health. The difference between sedentary level and active level has much to do with the increased calorie needs as well as increased protein needs associated with maintaining muscle mass. It is important to go for high quality proteins in the event that your diet involves moderate amounts of proteins. Therefore, you should be ingesting dairy products, eggs and meat, which consist of complex protein that your body requires. Low quality protein, such gelatin and collagen are found in low quality protein shakes. Ingesting a lot of protein is especially crucial in the first three weeks of a Ketogenic diet. When you get past the first three months of KD, you can significantly cut your protein intake if you feel you are consuming too much at that time.

3. Carbohydrate Intake

This is one of the most important aspects of the Ketogenic diet. The diet's main principle is dependent on the amount of carbs ingested in the body. Restricting the number of carbs that you ingest can easily get you into Ketosis. Instead of consuming any type of carbohydrate, you can opt to consume carbohydrates that are not linked with increased levels of insulin in the body. There are some specific types of carbs that can easily increase the blood sugar level of the dieter, such table sugar, rice cakes, some fruits, white rice and white bread. Foods that are low on the index include seeds, nuts, vegetables and whole grains. The foods that are low on the index have specific things in common, such as high in fibre, fat and protein. You can help keep your body in Ketosis by going for high-fibre carbohydrates. Another significant point to take into consideration is alcohol consumption. Alcohol is known to be harmful to a KD. This is so since most alcoholic products contain carbs; therefore, you might end up getting more calories than you might realize. In addition, alcohol can significantly inhibit Ketosis. If alcohol is part and parcel of your life then you should try as much as possible to minimize its consumption in order to get the most out of the Ketogenic diet.

Common Mistakes People Make When Undertaking The Ketogenic Diet

1. Keto Sticks

Most dieters on a KD use Keto sticks thinking that they will tell them what kind of state their bodies are in, and if they are in Ketosis or not. These are absolutely not accurate. The problem with Keto sticks is that if you drink a lot of water, you will have a diluted reading, so a light coloured reading. If you are dehydrated, you are going to have a dark color reading. So using these sticks does not determine how many Ketones you have in your blood at that time.

2. Unstable Glucose Levels

Fluctuating glucose levels are not good for your body either – it is not good for your body deciding what parts or fuel sources to utilize. Therefore, try as much as possible to keep the glucose levels stable. You can achieve stable glucose levels by reading your glucose with a glucometer. The best glucometer should be a precision extra. This model is good, because it does Ketones as well as glucose. Monitoring your glucose and observing what you are eating while maintaining the glucose at a good level is the best approach. A reading less than 4.4 mm/ol is good to maintain an optimal glucose level.

3. Too Much Food Protein

Dieters on KD assume that they can eat beef, chicken, bacon and eggs the whole day. Well, that is not the case. You should aim at eating 70 to 80 grams and you will still feel strong while exercising, feel great the whole day and have lots of energy. So don't think that you have to be eating 100-200 grams of protein, since you technically do not have to do that. All that excess protein the body converts into sugar in a process called gluconeogenesis. This is simply the metabolic process that forms glucose from non-carbohydrates, such as proteins. When sugar goes into your blood, you will be back into that vicious cycle once again. Therefore, do not eat too much protein. 70-80 grams is what you should eat as a general rule.

4. Eating Too Much

Most people think that they can eat a lot of food and they will be okay as long as they are not eating carbs. Well, this is very wrong indeed. You do not want to count calories, but you have to be cautious about what you are eating. Basically, be smart, and when you are smart, you are not going to overeat. When you start getting Ketosis, you start getting Keto-adapted. Your hunger will drop with time and you will not want to eat as much. In the long-term, it is going to be easier for you, so just be prepared to think and stick it out from the very beginning.

5. Not Eating Enough Fat

KD is a high fat diet, but people may have a fat phobia. People may be hesitant to eat too much fat, but that does not make sense. For the KD to be effective, you need to eat lots of fat. This means that 80% of your daily intake of macronutrients should be fat. A good example of good fats as discussed earlier in the book is coconut oil. How about avocado? Just pure avocado? This is great, you can make guacamole and many great things out of it and it tastes good. MCT oil, the best part of the coconut oil is in here, but coconut has a lot of nutrients in it. This is great as well, because it will give you the energy you need. You can use avocado oil for cooking and you can season it on your salad dressing. All these are great sources of fat. As far as meat is concerned, you want full fat meat such as full fat beef and regular ground beef. You can also go for chicken wings, that type of thing, and bacon of course. Therefore, do not buy chicken breast and low-fat since you will be not helping yourself. Keep it high-fat, you will stay full, you will have lots of energy and that is what you want.

6. Eating In-Excess of Carbohydrates

Another big mistake most people make when using the KD is consuming too many carbohydrates either directly or indirectly. The primary goal of KD is to reduce the body's dependence on carbs for energy and seek alternative sources through Ketosis. As discussed earlier, most people are challenged by the sources of carbs. There are so many processed foods that people eat that are not a good sources of carbs. Ketosis requires you to minimize as much as possible your carb intake in order for your body to produce plenty of Ketones. You should be extremely careful when drinking alcohol. Most alcoholic products are known to contain too many carbs.

Chapter 4 – What Recipes, Staples & Ingredients to Keep on Hand in Your Kitchen

Keto Breakfast Recipes

1. Scrambled Eggs with Balsamic Vinegar

This meal consists of scrambled eggs with balsamic vinegar.

Ingredients:

The recipe requires you to have the following ingredients: four whole eggs; one finely chopped small onion; one finely chopped small tomato; half teaspoon of red chili powder; two teaspoons of balsamic vinegar; one finely chopped teaspoon of fresh coriander; one tablespoon of butter; and low sodium salt and pepper to taste.

Preparation:

Heat half tbsp of butter in a large slippery pan. Then sauté the chopped onion until transparent and crack the eggs while adding them into the pan one after the other. Go ahead and add pepper, salt and oregano and cook until a little brown in color. Transfer the cooked eggs to serving plates. Then melt the rest of the butter and heat for a couple of minutes. Then stir in balsamic vinegar and cook for another one minute. Poor hot butter and add vinegar over cooked eggs and garnish with coriander leaves. Then serve the meal hot.

2. Crispy Chicken

This is a nutty breakfast of chicken wings coated with eggs and nuts mix.

Ingredients:

The recipe requires you to have: one chicken wing; one large egg; one teaspoon of grounded flax seed; one tsp. of almond flour; one tsp of grounded hemp nuts; one tbsp.. of extra-virgin olive oil; and low sodium salt and pepper to taste.

Preparation:

Beat the eggs with pepper and salt in a bowl. Add hemp nuts, ground flaxseed and almond flour in a zip bag and shake well. Heat the oil in a slippery frying pan by using medium heat. Coat the chicken wing with whisked egg and then put it in the bag dry mix, and shake well so that the chicken is evenly coated. Place the chicken wing in the pan and cook for three minutes on each side until done. Then serve hot.

3. Baked Meatballs with Yoghurt Dip

Ingredients for Meatballs:

The ingredients required are: one pound of ground beef; two tsps. of fresh rosemary; one tsp. of grated ginger; one tsp. of coriander powder; one tsp. of cumin powder; half tsp. of onion powder; half tsp. of ground Jamaica pepper; ¼ tsp. of paprika; ¼ tsp. of oregano; ¼ tsp. of curry powder; one tbsp. of freshly chopped fresh coriander leaves; and low sodium salt and pepper.

Ingredients for Yoghurt Dip:

The ingredients required are: half cup of Greek yoghurt; 1¼ tsp. of cumin powder; one tbsp. of finely chopped fresh coriander leaves; one tbsp. of finely chopped fresh mint; zest of ½ limes; one tsp. of lime juice; and ¼ tsp. of low sodium salt.

Preparation:

Start by preheating the oven to 350°F. Then in a large bowl, break the ground beef with your hands. Add pepper, salt, coriander leaves, curry powder, oregano, paprika, Jamaica pepper, onion powder, cumin powder, coriander powder, ginger and rosemary to the beef. Then again mix the ingredients so that the spices are well distributed. Create eighteen to twenty balls from the beef. Once you made the balls, lightly grease a cookie sheet with olive oil and place the meatballs in it and then bake for fifteen minutes. Then mix the yoghurt, cumin powder, coriander leaves and mint in a bowl. Then again stir, add lemon zest, salt and lemon juice and mix well. Let the meatballs cool for a few minutes before serving. Once the meatballs have cooled, serve warm with faux yogurt sauce on side.

4. Bacon Soufflé with Swiss Cheese and Greek Yogurt

Ingredients:

The ingredients you need are: six ounces of finely chopped bacon; one small chopped onion; 1½ tsps. of grated garlic; six large eggs; one cup of shredded Swiss cheese; ½ cup of Greek yogurt; three finely chopped tablespoons of fresh coriander leaves; three tablespoons of extra-virgin olive oil; butter for greasing; and low sodium salt and pepper.

Preparation:

Preheat the oven to 400°F and lightly grease six ramekins. Heat the oil in a non-stick pan over medium heat and then sauté the onion until they are soft. Stir in the garlic and then continue cooking until the garlic turns somewhat brown. Get a large bowl and whisk eggs with pepper, salt, coriander and yogurt. Then again add olive oil, cheese and bacon and mix appropriately. Add sautéed onion and garlic and mix well. Pour the mix equally into prepared ramekins and bake for twenty minutes. Allow the meal to cool and serve warm.

5. Tuna Burger with Scrambled Eggs

Ingredients:

This recipe requires you to have: ½ pound of canned tuna; two tablespoons of minced onion; three ounces of cream cheese; three large eggs; one tablespoon of butter; low sodium salt and pepper.

Preparation:

Melt half tablespoon of butter in a large slippery pan over medium heat. Then sauté the onions with tuna in the pan until turn brown. Once turned brown, stir in the cheese and cook over low heat until melted, remove from the heat and transfer to a bowl and let it cool. Melt the remaining butter over medium heat. Whisk the eggs with pepper and salt, and then pour the whisked eggs into the pan and scramble until done. Come up with four flat round patties of cooked tuna about ½ inch thick. Then again place the patties in a serving plate, put scrambled eggs over two of the patties and cover with remaining two patties like a burger. Once done, serve immediately.

6. Pumpkin Pie Spiced Waffles

Ingredients:

This recipe requires the following ingredients: ½ cup of almond flour; two tablespoons of flaxseed meal; 1/3 cup of coconut milk; a quarter cup of canned pumpkin; 1½ tablespoons of pumpkin pie spice; one teaspoon of vanilla extra; one teaspoon of baking powder; two large eggs; three tablespoons of swerve sweetener; and seven drops of liquid stevia.

Preparation:

Mix all the ingredients in a sizeable measuring jug. Stir to mix the ingredients appropriately until there is little visibility of egg white. Add the dry components to a sifter. Then again sift all the dry components into the wet components. Combine the butter with the rest of the ingredients until all mix well. Have your waffle maker greased with coconut oil and then decant the batter onto the waffle. Set your waffles to bake and when they are ready serve with a few pecans and some maple syrup.

Keto Main Recipes

1. Keto Cobb Salad

This is a unique as well as delicious salad, which contains healthy proteins and fats for dieters on KD.

Keto Cobb Salad Ingredients:

The required ingredients for the salad include: two slices of turkey bacon; a hundred grams of ham; ½ diced avocado; extra-virgin olive oil; four cherry tomatoes; two cups of coarsely chopped romance lettuce; two hard-boiled eggs; and thirty grams of blue cheese.

Dressing Ingredients:

The ingredients required are: salt, pepper, a small amount of garlic, one tsp. of Dijon Mustard, one tsp. of lemon juice, one tbsp. of organic apple cider vinegar, and one tbsp. of extra-virgin olive oil.

Keto Cobb Salad Preparation:

Start by hard boiling the eggs using the regular technique. Have the ham sliced into cubes and then heat them in a pan pasted with olive oil for at least 3 minutes. Go ahead and cut the hard-boiled eggs. Have the lettuce placed at the bottom of a bowl. Place ontop the turkey bacon, eggs, ham, blue cheese, avocadoes and halved cherry tomatoes. Once you are done, go ahead and apply the dressing evenly. Then serve.

This Keto meal is highly nutritional as far as macronutrients are concerned. Macro nutrients obtained from the meal are 67% fat, 25% proteins and 8% carbs.

2. Keto Ground Beef Styr Fry

This is just the recipe one needs when under the Keto diet, because it does not only boost the immune system, but also the metabolism.

Ingredients:

The required ingredients are: one tablespoon of coconut oil; ½ medium Spanish onion; five medium brown mushrooms; two leaves of kales; ½ cup of broccoli; ½ medium red pepper; three hundred grams of ground beef; one tablespoon of Chinese five spices; and one tablespoon of Cayenne pepper.

Preparation:

Chop up the kales, onion, red pepper, broccoli and mushrooms. Go ahead and heat the coconut oil over medium heat in a big skillet and then add onions for at least 60 seconds. Mix the rest of the vegetables and then cook for another 2 minutes while stirring every now and then. Go ahead and add the spices and ground beef and cook for 1 1/2 minutes and then reduce the heat. Have the skillet covered and allow it to cook until the meat color turns brown. Then serve and enjoy this delicious Keto meal.

3. Fat Burning Ginger Beef

Ginger beef is one of the best Ketogenic diet recipes that anyone who is serious about Ketosis should try.

Ingredients:

You need the following ingredients for this recipe: a small amount of salt & pepper; four tbsps. of apple cider vinegar; one tbsp. of ground ginger; two small diced tomatoes; one crushed clove garlic; one small diced onion; one tbsp. of olive oil; and two sirloin steaks.

Preparation:

Have the oil placed in a large frying pan and heat the steaks over medium-high heat. Add the tomatoes, garlic, and onion the moment both sides of the steaks are seared. Get a bowl and combine a mixture of vinegar, pepper, salt and ginger. Then add the mixture to the frying pan and stir. Reduce the heat to low and cover the frying pan and allow the meal to simmer. Once all the liquid has evaporated, serve and enjoy your ginger beef.

4. Low Carb Chicken Salad

This is a good source of macronutrients as far as the KD is concerned.

Ingredients for the Salad:

The salad requires the following ingredients: ½ cup of sliced green onion; ½ cup of diced celery; and two cups of chicken.

Ingredients for the Dressing:

The dressing requires the following ingredients: salt & pepper; ½ teaspoon of dried thyme; one teaspoon of dried tarragon; three ounces of mayonnaise; and three ounces of softened cream cheese.

Preparation:

Mix all the salad ingredients along with the dressing. Then serve.

5. Low-Carb Baked Salmon

Ingredients:

The required ingredients are: two pounds of salmon fillets; four ounces of sesame oil; ½ cup of tamari soy sauce; one tsp. of minced garlic; ½ tsp. of ground ginger; ½ tsp. of basil; one tsp. of oregano leaves; ¼ tsp. of thyme; ½ tsp. of rosemary; ¼ tsp. of tarragon; four ounces of butter; half cup of fresh chopped mushrooms; and half cup of green chopped onions.

Preparation:

Combine the spices, sesame oil and tamari sauce and then pour into a Ziploc bag. Add the salmon to this sauce in the bag and refrigerate. Pre-heat the oven to 350°F and line a large frying pan with foil. Pour the marinade and salmon into the frying pan. Bake the fillet for at least ten minutes. Make sure the veggies are ready in time as you bake the salmon.Heat up some butter. Once the salmon is read go ahead and add the butter mixture over the salmon filters. Just ensure that the individual fillets are covered sufficiently. Then bake it for at least ten minutes over 350°F heat and serve immediately. This meal will provide you with adequate macronutrients as far as your Keto program is concerned.

6. Low Carb Meatloaf

This recipe combines perfectness and a delicious taste to your Ketogenic diet plan, and it does not have binders or bland.

Ingredients:

The ingredients you require include the following: half cup of almond oil; half cup of grated dry Parmesan cheese; two tablespoons of butter; eight ounces of chopped white onion; five minced garlic gloves; one cup of chopped green pepper; two large eggs; one tablespoon of finely chopped fresh basil leaves; ¼ cup of fresh minced parsley leaves; one tablespoon of thyme leaves; one tablespoon of salt; half tablespoon of ground black pepper; two teaspoons of Dijon mustard; ¼ cup of heavy cream; two pound of ground beef; one pound of Italian sausage; and half teaspoon of unflavored gelatin.

Preparation:

Have the oven preheated to 350°F and then use butter to grease a sizeable baking dish. Obtain a small bowl and whisk Parmesan cheese and almond oil. Place butter in conveniently large frying pan and heat over medium heat. Then add pepper, garlic and onion and sauté for at least for eight minutes. Set this mix aside as you prepare the rest of the ingredients. You should then mince the veggies to fine consistency by running through a food processor. Obtain another bowl and whisk the eggs with cream, BBQ sauce, mustard, pepper, salt and spices. Go ahead and pour some gelatin over the mix and allow it to settle for at least five minutes.

Then add minced onions to the combination. Mix the sausage and beef ensuring that there are no unmixed hunks of sausage left. Add the egg blend to the meatloaf and mix well. The again add to the mix the almond flour. Make sure that you blend the mixture appropriately. Have the mixture placed in a glass baking dish. Bake the mixture over 160°F. The loaf should cook in approximately one hour and then cool for about twenty minutes. Slice the meat loaf and then serve. This meal should provide you with four hundred and nine calories, including: one gram of fiber; five grams of carbohydrates; twenty three grams of protein and thirty three grams of fat.

7. Butter-Paneer Chicken Curry

This is a very delicious meal for a dieter on Keto diet.

Ingredients:

This recipe requires you to have the following ingredients: five sprigs cilantro; half teaspoon of red chili powder; half teaspoon of Kashmiri mirch; half teaspoon of paprika; one teaspoon of ground black pepper; one teaspoon of salt; one teaspoon of Garam masala; one teaspoon of coriander powder; 1½ teaspoon of ginger paste; 1½ teaspoon of garlic paste; two teaspoons of coconut oil; one teaspoon of olive oil; four tablespoons of butter; ½ cup of whipping cream; one cup of crashed tomatoes; one cup of water; seven ounces of Paneer packet; and three pounds of chicken thighs.

Preparation:

Start by preheating your oven to 375°F. Apply olive oil to the chicken thighs and then add pepper and salt to taste. Place the chicken thighs on a cooking sheet and allow them to roast for twenty five minutes. Carefully slice the Paneer into sizeable pieces. Place coconut oil and butter on a frying pan and heat over medium heat, allowing the butter to turn brown. Then again, add garlic paste and ginger to the brown butter for at least two minutes. Go ahead and pour into the pan the crushed tomatoes.

Then add salt, red chili powder, paprika, Garam masala, and coriander powder and mix and simmer. Carefully add the Paneer to the sauce. Go ahead and add water and allow the mixture to simmer for at least five minutes. Maintain medium low heat and pour in cream and stir. Allow the mixture to simmer for a while. Add the chicken thighs to the sauce and mix accordingly. Let the mixture simmer for about five minutes. Finally, garnish the mixture with cilantro and then serve.

Keto Desserts

1. Low-Carb Coconut Macaroon

Ingredients:

You need: two ounces chocolate chips; two ounces white chocolate syrup; two ounces heavy cream; eight ounces of softened cream cheese; sixteen ounces of unsweetened dried coconut; one cup erythritol; 1/8 teaspoon of salt; ¼ teaspoon of tartar cream; one teaspoon of vanilla; and four large egg whites.

Preparation:

Start by preheating your oven to 325°F. Then have cookie sheets lined in a large mixing bowl. In the bowl add salt, cream of tartar, vanilla and beat in the egg whites and mix to form tips curl. Add erythritol and fold in coconut. Then beat heavy cream and cream cheese until it is smooth. Then add syrup and coconut mixture and mix properly and fold in chocolate chips. Drop coconut blend in knolls on the cookie sheets you have prepared by using a small ice cream scoop. Have the mixture stored in an airtight container and let it stay for at least five days. Then go ahead and prepare fifty six cookies from the mixture.

2. Burrito

This is a low carb roll that is filled with cheese and salsa, vegetables and eggs.

Ingredients:

The ingredients required are: low sodium salt and pepper; half tablespoon of butter; shredded Mexican cheese blend; two flax seeds; two tablespoons of Mexican salsa; two whole organic eggs; two teaspoons of grated ginger; half teaspoon of red chili powder; ¼ cup of finely chopped tomato; ¼ cup of finely chopped onion; and ¼ cup of finely chopped green bell peppers.

Preparation:

Whisk eggs in a sizeable bowl and then add salt, pepper, chili powder, ginger, tomato, onion and bell pepper and mix appropriately. Melt butter in a large slippery pan over medium heat. Add the egg mix into the pan and scramble until done. Place tortillas in a serving place; put cooked eggs over tortillas shell and then top with cheese and salsa. Roll the tortillas gently into a tight coil. Then serve hot.

3. Brownie Cheesecake

Ingredients:

For the brownie base, you will need the following: ¼ cup of walnuts; ¼ teaspoon of vanilla; ¾ cup of granulated erythritol; two large eggs; pinch salt; ¼ cup of cocoa powder; ½ cup of almond flour; two ounces of unsweetened chocolate; and ½ cup butter.

For cheesecake filling, you will need: ½ teaspoon of vanilla extract; ¼ cup of heavy cream; ½ cup of granulated erythritol; two large eggs; and one pound of softened cheese.

Preparation:

Start by preheating your oven to 325°F and apply butter to your frying pan and then cloak the bottom of the pan with foil. Place chocolate and butter in a small pan and melt by placing over low heat. Whisk salt, cocoa powder and almond flour in a small bowl. Prepare the eggs by beating them in a large bowl and then add the almond flour mixture followed by butter and stir in nuts accordingly. Then spread the mixture over the pan you had initially prepared and bake for at least fifteen minutes. You should reduce your oven temperature to 300°F for the filling. For the filling obtain a large bowl and beat the following: eggs and cream cheese and vanilla. Place the filling over crust and then place your cheesecake on a sizeable cookie sheet. Go ahead and bake for thirty five minutes and allow cooling. Serve with chocolate sauce, which is sugar-free.

Chapter 5 – How to Start the Keto Diet

Nutritional Ketosis is Ketones that you use as small energy packs. Most people are engaging glucose as their energy pack. In nutritional Ketosis, you are by definition burning fat and a byproduct of burning fat is an energy pack that gives you profound energy at much greater levels than you get when you are burning carbs as your primary source. The human physiology is designed to exist on Keto and it is the way people have lived for seven thousand years.

Many people decides to launch into a Keto lifestyle head-on without understanding what they are getting into. Ketosis life is difficult, cravings are difficult and that is why most people do not engage in this lifestyle changing to a Keto diet, since it is just too difficult. In most parts of the world people usually live on a carb diet, which uses glucose as their principal fuel source instead of Ketones. The carbolic population is growing fast. There is a revolutionary new product introduced in the market, which is being referred to as the "*bridge to Ketosis*" – key Tobia. This brand new product allows dieters to get into Ketosis in one hour instead of nearly one week. You basically have to drink all natural drinks that launches the body into a state of Ketosis within an hour or two. What Key Tobia does is leverage your body to perform miracles and all it needs is a raw material.

Easy Steps to Start Eating a Keto Diet

To successfully start the Keto diet, you will have to start building your meals around good fats, such as avocados, extra-virgin oil and coconut products. These are foundational pieces for this nutritional plan. Also you can use grass-fed butter from grass fed cows, while raw cheese from grass-fed cows is another great source because you get tons of essential fats. Supplements such as fish oil, flaxseed oil or hemp oil are all good stuff too. You can use different seeds, such as sprouted chia seeds and hemp seeds. All these are loaded with really good fibre.

The KD is not a high protein diet. You certainly need some protein, but you need to source really clean animal sources. Therefore, grass-fed beef, which conserves key essential fats, such as omega 3 which are really powerful for your metabolism and they are contained in organic poultry and pasture-raised eggs. So eggs are phenomenal. A lot of people think that they want to consume only the egg white because they do not want the fat. However, the best part of the egg is the fats, the yolk is where all the anti-oxidants are. That is where the nutrients that fuel your brain and help your body adapt to Ketosis; they are actually in the yolks. You definitely want that that in your Keto diet. A lot of times people have issues of how to approach the Ketogenic diet. The perceptions are individualized for each person with respect to the carbohydrates load. It depends on what stage you are at and how physically active you are going to be.

Consume more liquids and more vegetables. Many people may perhaps think that they would get too hungry. But you can opt for intermittent fasting, where you eat your meals in six hour intervals. However, if someone has adrenal stress or major adrenal fatigue, they will not be able to do intermittent fasting effectively. Their energy is going to be really low without fuel and they are going to be burning through their adrenal hormones. Therefore, sometimes in those cases, you just need to prime your system with small amounts of proteins and good fats.

So perhaps you can try something like a half a can of organic coconut milk with maybe a scoop of either hypo-allergenic protein powder like a hemp protein or if you are not allergic use grass Steinway protein. Something small like the aforementioned provides something like fifteen to twenty grams of protein and about twenty to thirty grams of fat for every two hours to just keep the body running, while teaching the body to operate on Ketosis. There are usually two commonalities among individuals who get super hungry on Keto diets. The first is that they have issues with the basis of Ketosis regulations and secondly most have some type of stomach problems. If a dieter is not moving his bowels, then he or she is constipated. You know peristalsis or the muscle activity of the intestines helps to move the belly. Therefore, when you eat or anything going into the stomach, it helps stimulate peristalsis. So often times you might not be really hungry, but for whatever reason your body will give you signals to eat. The real message is that it wants the stimulants it is used to.

The Targeted Keto Diet and Workout

The principle of the diet is simple just consume some carbs before a workout in order to give your body a little extra fuel during a workout session to help your body synthesize glycogen after the workout. Technically, your body has enough fuel for training when you are on the Keto diet and in a state of Ketosis. Yet you will find it beneficial to have some carbs before training, which is a common variation for individuals who exercise regularly. As discussed earlier, twenty five to fifty grams of carbohydrates should make recovery from training easier and more comfortable.

If you are completing a very large amount of high-intensity training, you may want to have some carbohydrates during or after training. You should always remember to stick to simple and small amounts of carbohydrates in order to maintain the general principle of Ketosis. Depending on how hard you are working out and how many grams of carbohydrates you are consuming, you might be out of Ketosis for a very short time or a little longer. Because you only ingest carbs at specific times, you will maintain your state of Ketosis and burn through your fat store quickly.

Exercising To Maximize Weight Loss

Now that you understand how to go about the Keto diet, it is time to get a comprehensive idea of how you can use exercise to expedite your fat burning and improve your body composition. In addition to Ketosis and significant consumption of carbs before a training session, you will experience the following health benefits. Just make sure that you choose an exercise that works for you. You should not add exercise to your diet by forcing yourself to do workouts that are too streneous. Do something systematic that will help with your Ketogenic diet. For instance, you can walk, jog or a simply play tennis.

Cardiovascular Benefits

Workouts tax your heart, circulatory system and lungs, making them stronger over time. This helps to avoid cardiovascular disorder. The preventative effects come about mainly through a reduction of your blood pressure and an improvement in your good cholesterol to bad cholesterol ratio. Workouts may also improve the ability of your blood vessels to dilate when required, helping to get oxygen to your muscles when needed most.

Musculoskeletal Benefits

It is beneficial to use your muscles on regular basis even if you are undertaking a Keto diet. It has all types of benefits in everyday life. As you age, you will tend to lose your muscle mass, and by building up your muscles before this starts taking place, you will be able to continue doing regular activities later in your life without any difficulties.

Conclusion

The Ketogenic diet was initially been designed to treat epileptic patients. However, over the years, research has clearly indicated that this is one of the best diets you can implement to lose weight. There are many challenges associated with this diet, but they simply that, challenges, not obstacles. One of the major challenges is abandoning high carb diets to engage a Keto diet that is based on high fat intake. Ketosis, as discussed in the book is a very unique process of getting rid of fats out of the body. The book has elaborated the importance of Ketosis and how one can go about doing it the right way over a sustainable period of time. There are various benefits associated with Ketosis, including: reduced heart disease, lower blood pressure, reduced blood sugar and of course weight loss. Therefore, if you want to lose weight by burning fat get on the Keto diet NOW!